Brazilian Butt Lift

Your Guide to Achieving the Best Long-Term Results

WILLIAM R. BURDEN
M.D., F.A.C.S.

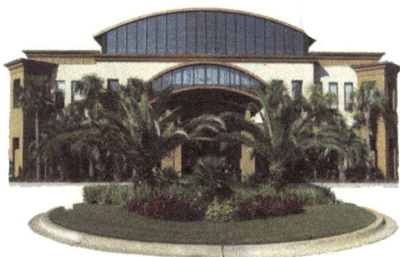

DESTIN
PLASTIC SURGERY
www.ThePlasticDoc.com

Published by William R. Burden, M.D., F.A.C.S., Destin, Florida.

ISBN: 978-0-692-17113-4

This book is not intended for use as a source of medical advice. The information in this book is intended to provide basic information on Brazilian Butt Lift procedures and the subjects discussed. It is not intended to be comprehensive by any means. **This book is not intended to diagnose or to treat any medical conditions, or to replace the advice of the reader's physician(s).**

The reader should regularly consult a physician in matters related to his or her health, specifically with respect to any symptoms that may require diagnosis or medical attention. For diagnosis or treatment of any medical problems, consult your physician(s).

The author and publisher are not responsible or liable for any damages or negative consequences from any treatment, action, application or preparation to any person reading or following the information in this book.

While all attempts have been made to verify information provided in this publication, the author and publisher assume no responsibility for errors, omissions or contrary interpretation of the subject matter herein. Any perceived slights of specific persons or organizations are unintentional.

REVOLVE™ System and its design are trademarks of LifeCell Corporation, an Allergan® affiliate. Any other trademarks mentioned in this book are listed for reference purposes only and are the property of the respective trademark owners.

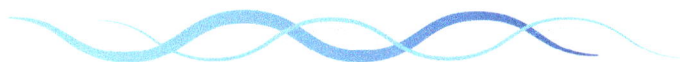

Table of Contents

Introduction   1

Questions and Answers   7

Before and After Pictures   25

What Patients Are Saying   29

About the Author   33

Glossary   41

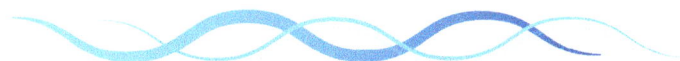

Introduction

This book is intended to be an overview of the Brazilian Butt Lift for women considering this procedure to enhance their buttocks. Although there are alternative procedures for buttocks enhancement, I believe the Brazilian Butt Lift, especially when incorporating the REVOLVE™ System, has the highest rate of satisfaction for patients when performed by a qualified plastic surgeon.

Buttocks Enhancement

Celebrities like Jennifer Lopez and Kim Kardashian are known for their hourglass figures, and more and more women are enquiring about enhancing their buttocks.

Procedures have been available for a few decades to obtain this result and historically, buttock implants were, and still are, used to add volume to this area. Although buttock implants are quite popular in South

America and some areas of the United States, use of implant placement is not free of problems.

Another technique, which we have used at Destin Plastic Surgery for some time, is grafting of the patient's own fatty tissue, or adipose, into the buttocks. This procedure has become known by the popular name, "The Brazilian Butt Lift". Although this procedure has been performed in The United States and Europe for many years, the Brazilians popularized it. The name has a nice sound to it and brings up an image of thong-clad women walking along the beach in Rio de Janeiro.

The ideal person undergoing a Brazilian Butt Lift has a little excess adipose of the hips and thighs and/ or the abdomen. This adipose, or fat, is removed, or harvested, using special techniques to maintain the viability of the adipose cells. The adipose cells are then grafted into the buttocks using special micro-cannulas into the areas that have a "deficiency" of volume that are to be "enhanced."

The combination of these two procedures, liposuc-tion/fat harvesting and lipoinfiltration/fat grafting, achieves a two-fold result: the hips, abdomen, and thighs are smaller and shapelier and the buttocks are fuller and rounder.

All of our patients who have undergone this procedure remark how much better their clothes fit and how they can wear low-waisted slacks and jeans without having a "muffin top." Their buttocks fill out the seat of the pants much better and they also remark about the improved fit of their bathing suits. Ladies frequently tell us that their spouses and friends remark on how shapely they appear after the procedure.

Fat Grafting Background

Fat grafting has been attempted in plastic surgery for many years, but about 25 years ago fat grafting techniques were still very unreliable. As much as 70 percent of the fat that was transferred did not survive after the grafting process. This meant that many times patients had to go through multiple grafting procedures just to get a minimal or modest result.

During the 1980s and early 90s fat grafting procedures were revolutionized using the microcannula technique. With this technique small tubes of fat grafts are laid down and the surrounding tissue provides the needed blood supply to help the fat graft survive. About this time I used the microcannula technique with very good success for lip augmentation and facial rejuvenation.

In the mid-90s, I saw a young girl who was brought to the office by her parents for evaluation for fat grafting. She had fallen off the monkey bars at school and landed on her buttock, causing a severe contusion to the buttock. The "crush injury" resulted in the fat dying in the mid-buttock, leaving a groove on her buttock. She was very self-conscious about this, and the children teased her, as the groove was apparent even in her clothing. Her parents had brought her to me to see if there was anything that could be done to improve the shape and decrease the severity of the defect.

I used a modification of the microcannula technique and harvested the fat from her hips. Although my expectations were somewhat guarded, the result was very good.

With that result in mind, I thought about applying the technique to other areas of the body. As time progressed, I offered fat grafting to people for multiple areas of fat loss. The back of a women's hand frequently looks masculinized, as the fat between the tendons has atrophied. The fat grafting can give them a more youthful-looking appearance. Breasts that have areas of defects from surgeries or injuries can be grafted to improve the contours.

Older women frequently asked me about augmentation in the lower buttock. Frequently, as women age they lose some of the fullness in their lower buttocks, especially in the area where they sit. I began doing fat grafting to the area, again achieving good-to-excellent results. As experience was gained, the grafting to the buttocks was expanded to cover not only replacing deficits but also enhancing the shape of the buttocks.

Early on, fat grafts were obtained with syringe liposuction and the fat grafts were purified using multiple techniques. Centrifuge, gravity filtration, and filter systems were used with increasingly good results.

Advanced Process for Improved Patient Satisfaction

In recent years an improved process for aesthetic and reconstructive fat grafting has been developed. The REVOLVE System is an integrated device that harvests, filters, and concentrates the fat tissue for grafting. I was very pleased with the results of fat grafts obtained using this system and I decided to start using it for grafts for buttocks augmentation. Patient benefits include a higher percentage of graft tissue remaining after recovery and an easier recovery without fluid leaking and draining.

Questions and Answers (Q&A's)

Q: What are the typical reasons that women consider having a Brazilian Butt Lift procedure?

A: The typical image, when we think of a patient considering a Brazilian Butt Lift, is a young lady who wants to have that real tiny waist and the full behind. In my experience that's not really the typical patient. Most patients want a fuller behind, but not necessarily an exaggerated appearance. For the majority of patients that I see, it's for a better fit in their clothes. They want to look good whether in casual or professional clothes as well as in their bathing suits.

A Brazilian Butt Lift can be a great solution because it can slim certain areas, like the hips, thighs, or abdomen, while increasing the volume in the buttocks area.

Women of all ages may be able to benefit from a Brazilian Butt Lift. When a woman reaches the age of 50 and over, she will commonly lose some of the fat in her buttocks. If we can take some of the fat she might have in her hips, tummy, or thighs and transfer it, she'll enjoy the fact that she doesn't have that saggy, droopy behind and her clothes fit much better. This is really noticeable in a bathing suit and the patients are very pleased because they can get their youthful figure back and they can fit much better in their clothes.

A Brazilian Butt Lift might be right for you if:

- You want a more curvy shape
- Your buttocks have a deficit of volume or have diminished or flattened over time
- Your clothes are not fitting well – the waist is tight and the area around the buttocks is loose
- You've gone through a massive weight loss or gastric bypass surgery and the buttocks volume is greatly diminished and the hips and back remain relatively large

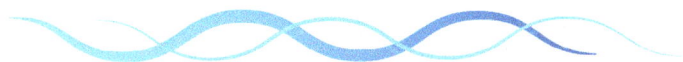

Q: Who are good candidates for a Brazilian Butt Lift?

A: Like with most plastic surgery procedures, a good candidate is a woman who's in overall good health, is in reasonably good shape, and has reasonable expectations for her results. She has a deficit of volume in her buttocks and is a little larger than she prefers in her hips, thighs, or abdomen. We will be harvesting fatty tissue from areas of excess, so we will slim down certain areas, while increasing the volume of the buttocks.

This procedure is not recommended for smokers. Smoking will decrease the blood supply, which will result in loss of the fat grafts, compromising the result. If the patient can quite smoking before the procedure and not start smoking again until approximately six weeks after, this will likely not be an issue, but patients are advised to discuss their particular situation regarding smoking with their surgeon during a pre-surgery consultation.

Potential patients that can benefit from a Brazilian Butt Lift include women from their mid-twenty's until well later in life. We can generally separate potential patients by age group along with characteristics we observe that are common at different stages in life.

25 to 35-year-old
The typical patient in this group either has a buttocks deficit or wants a more curvy shape. She has some areas she would like to slim such as hips, thighs, or abdomen, so we transfer fat cells from these areas and the result is a curvy shape.

35 to 45-year-old
Typically the patient has lost some of her buttocks volume and has developed larger hips after having children and getting older. The clothes are not fitting well.

45-55-year-old
Frequently the buttocks volume is moderately diminished and hip volume is enlarged. The lower buttocks, especially where they sit, is flattened. Clothes are not fitting well – the waist is tight and the area around the buttocks is loose.

55-75-year-old
The buttocks volume has typically moderately-to-severely diminished, but there is some excess volume in

hips, thighs, or abdomen. The lower buttock, espe-cially where they sit, is flattened. The upper buttock is enlarged, creating an inverted shape. Clothes are not fitting well - lots of nice dresses that they have in their closet don't fit well or like they once did.

Another candidate for the procedure is a patient that has gone through a massive weight loss of one hundred or more pounds or after a gastric bypass procedure. After a large weight loss, a woman will commonly lose the fat in her buttocks, but will continue to hold onto some fat in the hips and back, possibly in the abdomen. The deficient volume of fat in the buttocks results in an odd-shaped figure and makes fitting into clothes difficult. When we take the fat from the hips, back, and abdomen, and transfer it to the buttocks, that patient can regain a more normal figure with a normal proportion buttocks and she can appreciate a better fit in her clothes.

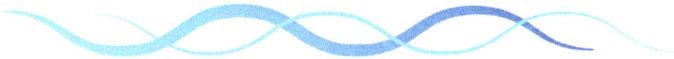

Q: What happens during the procedure?

A: The patient is taken to the operating room and treated very similar to a patient who's undergoing liposuction. In a Brazilian Butt Lift procedure, the fat is harvested using a suction that's not as harsh as we use with regular liposuction. We don't want to destroy the fat cells, so we want to gently remove them from the body so that we can then use them to graft back into the buttocks area. Fat cells are typically harvested from areas with excess fat, usually from the hips, thighs, abdomen, and/or back. The harvested fat cells are then rinsed and concentrated to remove fluids and cellular debris.

In my experience the manner in which the harvested fat cells are processed prior to injection is a key factor in the accurate grafting and shaping of the buttocks. For this reason, I use the REVOLVE System because it does a better job in removing excess fluids and other debris, concentrating the fat cells and making the grafts more viable. Another benefit is an easier recovery for the patient.

After the fat cells are processed, we precisely inject them into the buttocks using a microcannula.

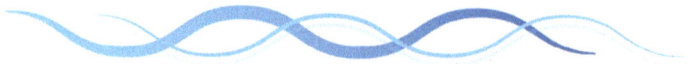

Q: What is the REVOLVE System?

A: The REVOLVE System is an innovative all-in-one, integrated device that harvests, filters, and concentrates adipose tissue. It is a sterile device that minimizes tissue handling and exposure to outside air and is typically used in aesthetic and reconstructive fat transfer procedures. The REVOLVE System is intended for single-use.

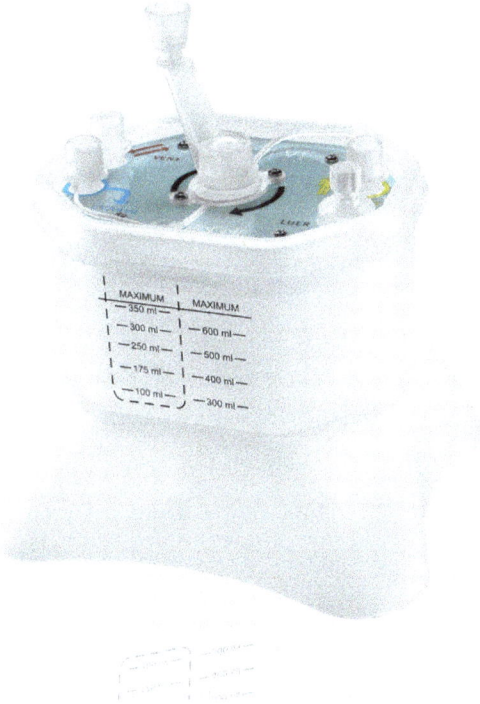

The REVOLVE™ System is a single-use, sterile device used for harvesting, filtering, and transferring of adipose tissue.

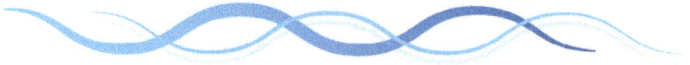

Q: Why does use of the REVOLVE System in a Brazilian Butt Lift procedure provide superior results and an easier recovery?

A: In a more conventional Brazilian Butt Lift procedure performed by most surgeons, the adipose being transferred has a lot of fluids that have not been filtered out of the fatty tissue. As a result, a significant amount of the total volume transferred is absorbed into the body or will drain out. Typically, only a fraction of the fat graft volume injected into the buttocks remains after the recovery.

With the conventional method, the incisions from the procedure are left open to allow the fluid that is not absorbed by the body to drain out. The drainage of that extra fluid that has been injected along with the adipose is very messy and can get on the sheets and towels that are laid on the bed during the recovery period.

Using the REVOLVE System, most of the fluid is filtered out and more concentrated fat grafts are placed, so we achieve a greater take of the grafts and require less volume to inject. With this method we don't leave the incisions open, so the patient doesn't have fluid leaking and draining out in the postoperative period.

One of my Brazilian Butt Lift patients has a friend that went to Miami for her Brazilian Butt Lift procedure. During her friend's procedure 1500ccs of fat grafts were injected; however, only approximately 800ccs took after recovery. Her friend also reported that while she was recovering, the incisions were left open and much of the fluid drained out onto her sheets and bed. In fact, her surgeon had told her to lay down towels to catch the fluid as it leaked out of the incisions.

By contrast, my patient had 900ccs transferred into each buttock and I estimate approximately 800ccs remained after she had recovered. My patient was very impressed that her incisions were closed and no fluid leakage occurred during her postoperative period. She felt that her friend had experienced a very messy first couple of days following her surgery.

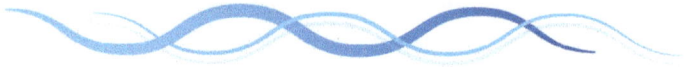

Q: What is the recovery like for your patients after a Brazilian Butt Lift procedure?

A: Patients generally are very swollen and bruised for approximately two to three weeks. They will be wearing a surgical support garment that compresses their waist and thighs but does not put as much pressure on the buttocks. That garment is usually worn for three weeks. After three weeks they can continue to wear it if they like, or switch to something that's not quite as stiff. Patients typically wear a Spanx or other softer compression garment for 3 more weeks.

After the procedure, patients are asked to lie on their side or their stomach and not put pressure on their buttocks. For those people who are back sleepers, we recommend that they either buy an egg-crate mattress and they cut a hole out for their buttocks to lie into. The egg-crate mattress will support their back and thighs. Alternatively, they can place pillows under their back and under their thighs and make a little trough for their buttocks. That will allow them to sleep without putting a lot of pressure on the areas that have been grafted. Also, when they are sitting, either at home or when they go back to work, they need to use a special pillow that goes under their thighs that takes the pressure off the buttocks, or use a donut-shaped pillow so that their buttocks sit in the donut and the pressure is applied to their thighs and the sides of their buttocks. Avoidance of pressure to the buttocks should be followed for 6 weeks after surgery.

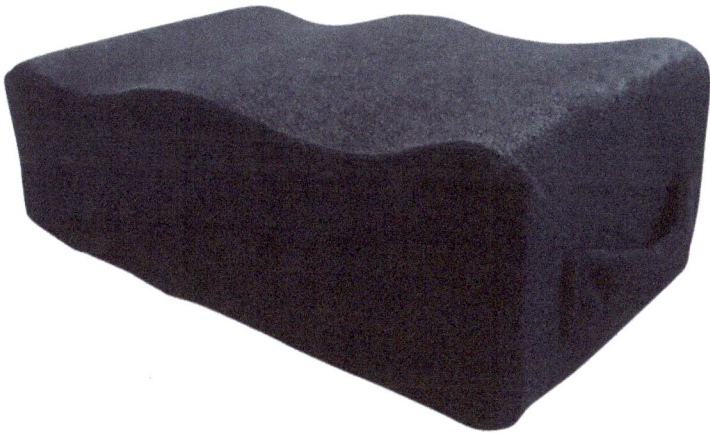

Booty Buddy® Support Cushion

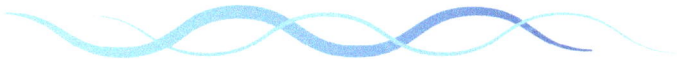

Q: When will the patient be able to go back to work and do some physical activity?

A: Most patients can get back to work in a matter of a week to 10 days. When they go back to work, they have to be very cautious not to sit down and apply a lot of pressure to their buttocks. Most of our patients who have desk jobs will stand or they'll get a special pillow that applies the pressure only to their thighs so that they don't put as much pressure on their buttocks. Patients who are physically active generally don't go back to work until day 10 to 14, as they will be sore in their hips, back, abdomen, and/or thighs, the areas where the fat has been harvested. In around two to three weeks, they'll feel comfortable doing light physical activity. Patients that typically are very physically active, like fitness instructors or who work very physical jobs, should be able to get back to their full activity level in about four to five weeks.

Q: Will there be a visible scar after the procedure?

A: There will be small scars, but they are well hidden in the crease under the buttocks and just beneath the sacral area. Sometimes we might have to put a scar in the inside of the umbilicus or in the groin region. These scars heal very well, are small (only about three to four millimeters in length), and are usually not very visible.

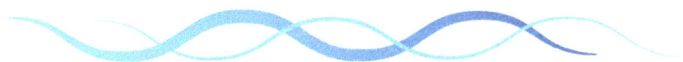

Q: How long will the results last?

A: If a patient maintains her diet and exercise regimen, she'll maintain the results for many years. As people age, they tend to lose a little fat in their buttocks and may gain a little fat in their hips and back. They may see those changes occur over time. Of course, if they maintain a good diet and exercise regimen, they'll maintain their results longer.

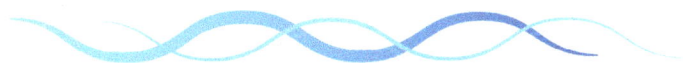

Q: If a patient has a job that requires sitting for up to eight hours per day, will that be an issue for long-term results?

A: Many of the patients we see in their 40s or 50s have already had a loss of fat and a little flattening in the area right over the ischium where they sit down. That's pretty typical because as people age they get a little flattening in that area. After they've fully recovered, patients who sit a lot will continue to lose some of the fat in their buttocks over time, but my patients who have desk jobs have been very pleased with their results over time.

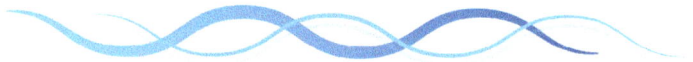

Q: If a patient continues to exercise after the procedure, and loses weight, will she lose the fat that has been grafted in her buttocks?

A: When a person loses weight, the loss of fat is proportional to the amount of fat cells located in the different parts of the body, so all of the areas of fat in the body will shrink. After losing weight, the buttocks will be fuller than if they had not had a Brazilian Butt Lift.

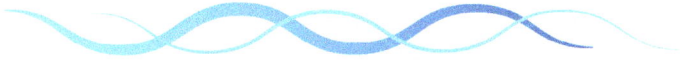

Q: Surgery in general has risks. What are some risks specific to the Brazilian But Lift surgery?

A: As with any surgery, there is a risk of infection, but it is very low. My surgeries are performed in an operating room with a very well maintained sterile environment. To date, my patients have not experienced an infection with this procedure.

Although not typically considered a complication, decreased survival of the fat grafts may result in a smaller increase to buttock volume.

I follow guidelines outlined in the literature to avoid fat embolism. To date, we have had no fat embolism results.

Q: Can a Brazilian Butt Lift be combined with other procedures?

A: Some patients interested in other procedures may want to combine procedures so their downtime and recovery are simultaneous. A Brazilian Butt Lift can be combined with other procedures like breast augmentation, a breast lift, or abdominoplasty (tummy tuck).

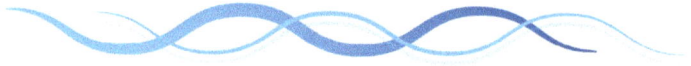

Q: Are there alternatives to a Brazilian Butt Lift, such as implants?

A: Implants have been used for many years for buttocks enhancement, but they are not without problems. Implants can be undesirably obvious and many patients complain that the implants are hard and very uncomfortable to sit on. Another common complaint relates to the scars from the incisions required to place the implants that extend from the sacral area to the crease between the buttocks. There are also risks of developing fluid around the implants, as well as infections, either of which would require removal of the implants.

For women who don't have adequate fat to transfer, an implant can be an alternative. When a patient is considering having implants, they should understand that the recovery is going to be a little more difficult. It's a painful recovery that can take two to three weeks.

Q: If a woman is interested in a Brazilian Butt Lift procedure, how should she select a qualified plastic surgeon?

A: Some research can be done by asking friends for recommendations and searching the Internet for surgeons specifically experienced in this procedure. It's important to know the plastic surgeon's experience specifically with performing Brazilian Butt Lift procedures as well in fat grafting to other areas. Find out if this is a procedure that is routinely performed or if it just once or twice a year. Ask to see pictures of results of actual patients and testimonials from actual patients.

I've remarked earlier in this book about the benefits and patient satisfaction when a surgeon uses the RESOLVE System to harvest, filter, and concentrate the fat cells that will be injected into the buttocks. For an easier recovery and better results, I'd recommend asking if your surgeon uses the REVOLVE device in their procedures.

A good experience for the patient starts with having good communications and rapport with your surgeon. Your surgeon should provide a thorough understanding of the procedure and answer all of your questions. Make sure that you sense that you are compatible with your surgeon during your consultation.

Finally, make sure that your surgeon is Board Certified by the American Board of Plastic Surgeons.

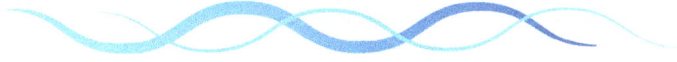

Before and After Pictures

On the following pages are **<u>actual</u>** before and after photos of four of Dr. Burden's Brazilian Butt Lift procedure patients.

Readers can see an extensive gallery of Dr. Burden's patients' before and after photos from various procedures by visiting:

https://www.ThePlasticDoc.com

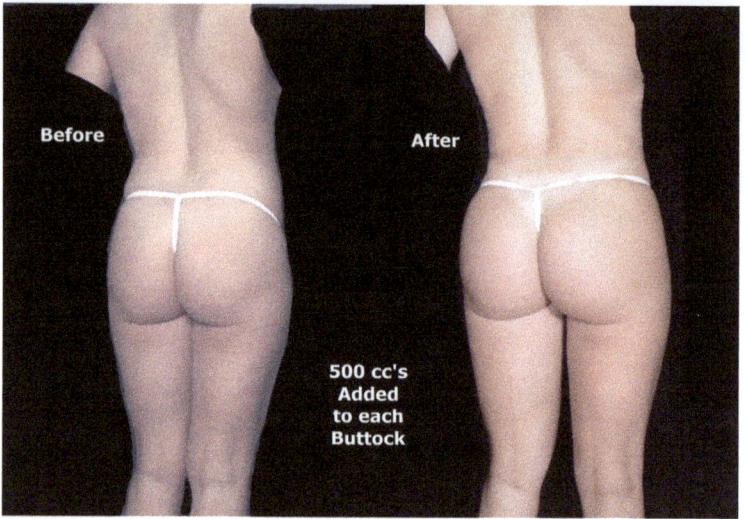

Before

After

500 cc's
Added
to each
Buttock

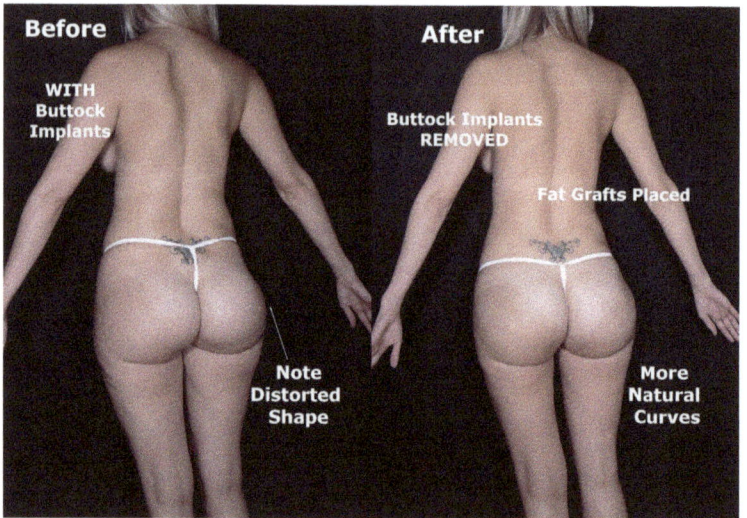

Before

After

WITH
Buttock
Implants

Buttock Implants
REMOVED

Fat Grafts Placed

Note
Distorted
Shape

More
Natural
Curves

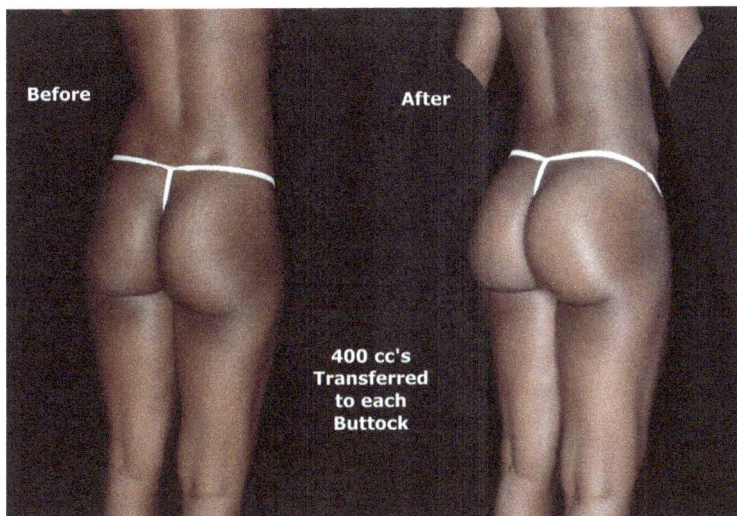

Before

After

400 cc's
Transferred
to each
Buttock

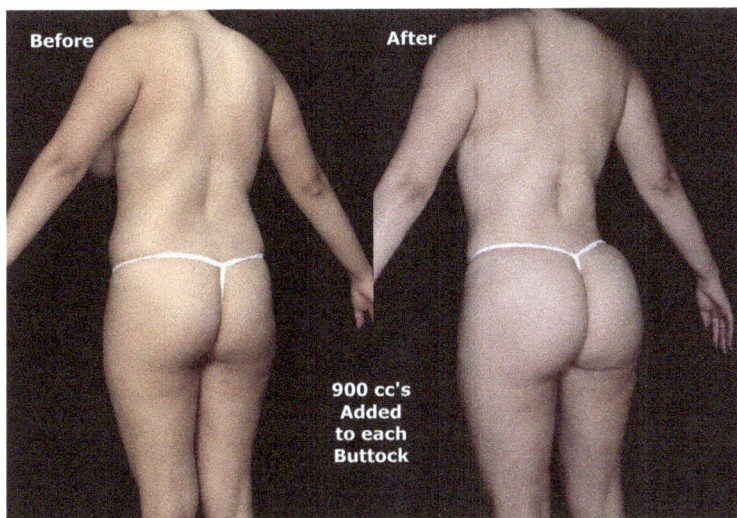

Before

After

900 cc's
Added
to each
Buttock

What Patients Are Saying

"As far as consult, pre-op, and day of surgery I am 100% happy with Dr. Burden and his whole staff. He is very kind, knowledgeable, compassionate, and does a great job of managing expectations. He has a very nice disposition, always smiling, you couldn't ask for a better Doc. Highly recommend, and if I ever chose to have another procedure done I would definitely return. Not a single negative thing to say about the whole experience."

"Day 1: So Far, So Good!!!!"

"PreOp visit was lovely, very professional and informative!!"

"So far, Dr. Burden is a very sweet and personable guy. He counseled me on my lifestyle after surgery such as eating habits and food choices. He took his time with me and wasn't in a rush at all. He didn't fast-talk me and used technology to show me the treatment areas and before/after effects. I like his nurse Joan and Machele (the payment rep). Joan gave me a list of meds and supplements to stay away from before surgery. I also left my pre op/consult with all my meds and orders for pertinent blood work. I'm excited to see what Dr. Burden does for me."

"The staff was great, answered all my questions, and kept in touch with me before and after. I even had 2 consults to make sure the doctor knew what I wanted."

"I've been considering BBL for about a year now. I have gained about 6 pounds for the surgery. Harvesting fat from back, flank, arms, inner thigh, abdomen. Aiming for a minimum of 1000 cc per cheek. He feels he can achieve this for me and will do his best to give me what I'm looking for! Feeling nervous yet positive. Tomorrow is the day! I'm going to do this as a way to keep busy..."

About the Author

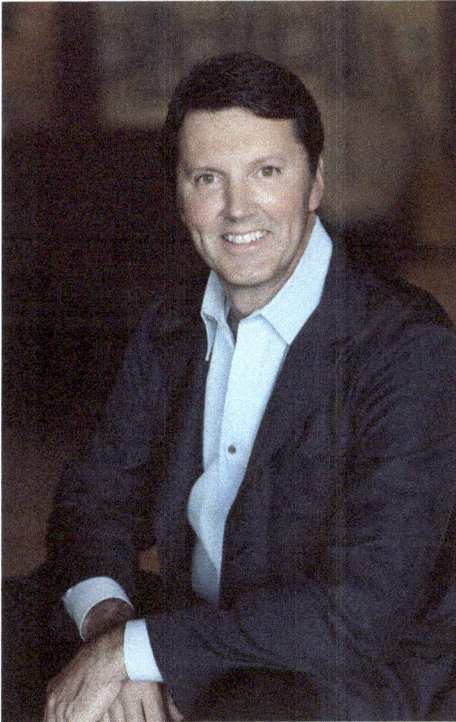

William R. Burden, M.D., F.A.C.S., is a Board Certified Plastic Surgeon, a Fellow of the American College of Surgeons and a member of the American

Society of Plastic Surgeons. He is the founder and CEO of Destin Plastic Surgery in Destin, Florida, one of the Southeast's most recognized cosmetic facilities. He is also the founder of the Destin Surgery Center, housed in the same building.

While in high school, Dr. Burden took anatomy classes offered at the Medical College of Virginia on the weekends. He also took classes in Medical Genetics and Computer programming. Because of high PSAT and SAT scores, he was selected to attend college classes prior to graduating from high school at Virginia Tech.

Dr. Burden received his Bachelor of Science in Biochemistry from Virginia Tech and his Medical Degree from the Medical College of Virginia. While at Virginia Tech, he was involved in genetics research. At the Medical College of Virginia, he was involved in Vitamin A research and its role in cancer prevention.

Dr. Burden completed his residency in General Surgery at Louisiana State University School of Medicine. While there, he authored several papers and was involved in vascular surgery research and spinal cord injury research.

While in his fellowship in Plastic Surgery at the University of Florida, Dr. Burden worked with his professors to introduce endoscopic techniques in breast surgery and specialized microvascular techniques for breast and body reconstruction.

During his fellowship at the University of Florida, Dr. Burden was one of the pioneers in researching the use of endoscopic or fiber optic technology for plastic surgery. He saw the potential for use of this new technology to enable accurate placement of breast implants using an incision in the underarm area instead of on the breast.

Dr. Burden's vision was to perfect a procedure using the latest technology that would provide the best results in terms of breast augmentation without leaving a visible scar on the breast. Although some breast augmentations had been done by plastic surgeons using an incision in the armpit prior to this time, the ability to accurately dissect and place the implants was a limiting factor in the use of this technique. During the course of his fellowship, Dr. Burden and the team he was working with were successful in achieving his vision.

When Dr. Burden entered private practice, he offered the transaxillary approach, with the incision in the armpit along with the more traditional approaches to breast augmentation. Even though all of the approaches to breast augmentation can provide good results in terms of breast volume and shape, over time, he found that the highest patient satisfaction level was achieved when the patient had no scar on the breast.

Dr. Burden is known nationally and internationally for the No Scar on the Breast procedure. He has been performing the No Scar on the Breast procedure for over twenty years and has completed thousands of No Scar on the Breast surgeries.

Women travel from across the country and from around the world to have their procedures performed by Dr. Burden. Among his patients are Miss USA and Miss America contestants, country music performers and bathing suit models, to mention a few. In addition to breast augmentation, Dr. Burden performs a full range of cosmetic and reconstructive surgical procedures on the face and body. He has appeared on news reports for his expertise with the Brazilian Butt Lift, facelifts, and eyelid surgery.

Dr. Burden has been on the Mentor Corporation advisory panel for both breast augmentation and breast reconstruction. He is also on the Allergan Corporation advisory panel for new technology in breast augmentation and for their facial aesthetics and injectables products. He is a member of the Allergan Speaker Bureau and instructs and educates other physicians, nurses, and medical personnel on facial aesthetic treatments. In addition, he has participated in the national study for the reintroduction of the silicone gel implant.

Dr. Burden has been added to a panel of surgeons advising plastic surgeons on the use of the REVOLVE system to improve the results of fat grafting. The surgeons on this panel are experienced with fat grafting to enhance the appearance on areas of the body including the face, breasts, buttocks, hands, and other areas needing contouring.

Dr. Burden's surgeries are conducted at the Destin Surgery Center, co-located with Destin Plastic Surgery. The center is fully accredited by the Accreditation Association for Ambulatory Health Care and was ranked as one of the best hospitals by *US News and World Report*. Over 30,000 procedures have been performed at this facility. A full-time attending anesthesiologist is the Medical Director of Destin Surgery Center.

For More Information

For more information about Dr. William Burden, the Brazilian Butt Lift, and other cosmetic procedures, visit:

https://www.ThePlasticDoc.com

Contact Information

Destin Plastic Surgery
The Grant Building
4485 Furling Lane
Destin, Florida 32541

Phone: (850) 654-1194
Toll-free: (866) ENHANCE (364-2623)

Glossary

Adipose: Fatty tissue that is located beneath the skin and around internal organs. Excess adipose, usually located in the hips, thighs, abdomen, and/or back, is harvested and transferred to the buttocks during a Brazilian Butt Lift procedure.

Brazilian Butt Lift (or BBL): A plastic surgery procedure in which fat is removed from areas of excess, such as the hips, thighs, abdomen, and/or back, and is precisely re-injected into the patient's buttocks to enhance the contour, size and/or shape of the buttocks. In addition to the enhancement of the buttocks, the patient will realize slimming of areas where the fat was removed.

F.A.C.S.: F.A.C.S. is an abbreviation that stands for Fellow of the American College of Surgeons.

Fat Grafting: The plastic surgery process of removing fat cells from areas of excess through liposuction and re-injecting the fat cells in areas where enhancement is desired. Also known as "fat transfer."

Fat Harvesting: The plastic surgery process of removing fat cells from areas of excess through liposuction prior to fat grafting. When liposuction is performed for the purpose of harvesting fat cells for grafting, the process is much gentler than ordinary liposuction to improve the viability of the fat cells being transferred.

Fat Transfer: The plastic surgery process of removing fat cells from areas of excess through liposuction and re-injecting the fat cells in areas where enhancement is desired. Also know as "fat grafting."

Implants (for Buttocks): Implants, usually made of semi-solid silicone, which are surgically inserted into the buttocks to enhance the size and shape of the buttocks. This is an alternative and now much less frequently performed procedure than a Brazilian Butt Lift.

Lipoinfiltration: Injection of the fat grafts into the soft tissues of the body typically performed to enhance the size and shape of an area or to improve the contour of a defect from an injury or surgery.

Liposuction: A plastic surgery procedure that removes fat from areas of the human body to change the shape of treated areas. During a Brazilian Butt Lift procedure, fat cells are removed from areas of excess through liposuction and the fat cells are filtered and concentrated before precisely re-injecting the fat cells into the buttocks to achieve enhancement. An additional result is the slimming of areas where the fat was removed.

Microcannula: A very small tube that is used to precisely re-inject fat cells into the area that is being enhanced.

REVOLVE™ System: An all-in-one, single-use, integrated device that harvests, filters, and concentrates fat cells. It is a sterile device that minimizes tissue handling and exposure to outside air and is typically used in aesthetic and reconstructive fat transfer procedures.

Notes

Notes

Notes

www.ingramcontent.com/pod-product-compliance
Lightning Source LLC
Chambersburg PA
CBHW042312210326
41598CB00041B/7361